MIND DIET COOKBOOK

Nutritious Recipe to Enhance Brain Function
and Prevent Memory Loss For
Alzheimer's Patient

LAKEISHA   OWENS

TABLE OF CONTENT

INTRODUCTION

Alzheimer's disease, a progressive neurological disorder that leads to memory loss and cognitive decline, affects millions of individuals and their families worldwide. Recent studies and clinical observations have increasingly highlighted the significant role that nutrition plays in not only managing but potentially mitigating the progression of Alzheimer's disease. It is within this context that the "MIND DIET COOKBOOK" emerges as an essential guide, aiming to provide nutritious and tailored recipes that cater specifically to the needs of those living with Alzheimer's, as well as preventive measures for those seeking to maintain brain health and mitigate risk factors associated with this condition.

Our journey through the pages of this cookbook is not merely about the act of cooking. It is an exploration of how food connects to memory, well-being, and the management of Alzheimer's symptoms.

We delve into the science of nutritional neuroscience and geriatric nutrition, presenting a collection of recipes rich in antioxidants, omega-3 fatty acids, vitamins, and minerals known to support brain health. Each recipe is crafted with simplicity in mind, considering the varying abilities and dietary needs of individuals at different stages of Alzheimer's disease.

As we embark on this culinary journey, our aim is to arm readers with knowledge, inspiration, and practical tools to navigate the complexities of Alzheimer's disease through the power of nutrition. Whether you are a caregiver, a loved one, or someone interested in brain health, the "Mind Diet Cookbook" invites you to explore the profound connection between what we eat and how we think, feel, and remember.

BREAKFAST RECIPE

RECIPES

BREAKFAST RECIPE

Blueberry & Spinach Smoothie

Ingredients:

1 cup fresh blueberries
1 cup baby spinach
1 banana
½ cup unsweetened almond milk
1 tablespoon flaxseeds

Instructions:

Blend all ingredients until smooth.

Serve immediately.

Greek Yogurt Parfait

Ingredients:

1 cup Greek yogurt

½ cup mixed berries

¼ cup walnuts

A drizzle of honey

Instructions:

Layer yogurt, berries, and walnuts in a glass.

Drizzle with honey.

Avocado Toast on Whole Grain Bread

Ingredients:

1 ripe avocado

2 slices whole grain bread

Cherry tomatoes

Olive oil

Lemon juice

Salt and pepper

Instructions:

Mash the avocado and mix with a squeeze of lemon juice, salt, and pepper.

Spread on toasted bread and top with sliced cherry tomatoes and a drizzle of olive oil.

Egg & Veggie Muffins

Ingredients:

6 eggs

1 cup diced vegetables (bell peppers, onions, spinach)

½ cup shredded cheese

Salt, and Pepper

Instructions:

Whisk eggs and add vegetables and cheese.

Season with salt and pepper.

Pour into greased muffin tins and bake at 350°F for 20-25 minutes.

Sweet Potato & Kale Hash

Ingredients:

1 large sweet potato (diced)

1 cup kale (chopped)

1 onion (diced)

2 tablespoons olive oil

2 eggs

Salt and pepper

Instructions:

Sauté sweet potato and onion in olive oil until tender.

Add kale, cook until wilted.

Make two wells in the hash, crack an egg into each

Cover and cook until eggs are set.

Almond Butter & Banana Oatmeal

Ingredients:

½ cup rolled oats

1 cup almond milk

1 banana (sliced)

2 tablespoons almond butter

Cinnamon

Instructions:

Cook oats in almond milk.

Stirring occasionally.

Serve topped with banana, a dollop of almond butter, and a

sprinkle of cinnamon.

Cottage Cheese & Pineapple Bowl

Ingredients:

1 cup cottage cheese

½ cup diced pineapple

¼ cup sliced almonds

A drizzle of honey

Instructions:

Mix cottage cheese with pineapple and almonds.

Drizzle with honey before serving.

Baked Avocado Eggs

Ingredients:

2 avocados
Halved and pitted
4 eggs
Salt, and pepper
Chopped chives for garnish

Instructions:

Place avocado halves in a baking dish, crack an egg into each half.

Season with salt and pepper.

Bake at 425°F for 15-20 minutes.

Garnish with chives.

Broccoli & Feta Omelette

Ingredients:

2 eggs

1 cup chopped broccoli

¼ cup feta cheese

1 tablespoon olive oil

Salt, and pepper

Instructions:

Sauté broccoli in olive oil.

Whisk eggs and pour over broccoli.

Sprinkle feta cheese on top.

Cook until set, then fold and serve.

Pumpkin Seed & Cranberry Energy Bars

Ingredients:

1 cup rolled oats

½ cup pumpkin seeds

½ cup dried cranberries

¼ cup honey

½ cup peanut butter

Instructions:

Mix all ingredients and press into a lined baking dish.

Chill until firm, then cut into bars.

LUNCH RECIPE

LUNCH RECIPE
Salmon Salad with Mixed Greens

Ingredients:

4 oz grilled salmon

2 cups mixed greens

½ avocado (sliced)

¼ cup walnuts

2 tablespoons vinaigrette dressing

Instructions:

Toss mixed greens, avocado, and walnuts with vinaigrette.

Top with grilled salmon.

Turkey and Avocado Wrap

Ingredients:

1 whole grain tortilla

4 oz sliced turkey breast

¼ avocado (sliced)

Lettuce

Tomato

Mustard

Instructions:

Lay tortilla flat

Layer with turkey, avocado, lettuce, and tomato.

Add mustard, roll up, and serve.

Broccoli and Cheddar Soup

Ingredients:

2 cups broccoli (chopped)

1 onion (chopped)

2 cups vegetable broth

1 cup cheddar cheese (shredded)

1 cup milk

Olive oil

Salt, and pepper

Instructions:

Sauté onion in olive oil

Add broccoli and broth, simmer until tender.

Blend until smooth

Return to heat, add milk and cheese

Stirring until melted.

Season with salt and pepper.

Mediterranean Chickpea Salad

Ingredients:

1 can chickpeas (drained)

1 cucumber (diced)

1 bell pepper (diced)

¼ cup olives (sliced)

¼ cup feta cheese

2 tablespoons olive oil

Lemon juice

Salt, and pepper.

Instructions:

Combine chickpeas, cucumber, bell pepper, and olives.

Toss with olive oil, lemon juice, salt, and pepper.

Sprinkle with feta before serving.

Spinach and Mushroom Frittata

Ingredients:

4 eggs

1 cup spinach (chopped)

½ cup mushrooms (sliced)

¼ cup grated Parmesan

2 tablespoons olive oil

Salt, and pepper

Instructions:

Sauté mushrooms in olive oil

Add spinach until wilted.

Whisk eggs with Parmesan, salt, and pepper, pour over vegetables.

Cook until set, then broil until golden.

Baked Sweet Potato with Black Bean Salsa

Ingredients:

2 sweet potatoes

1 can black beans (drained)

1 avocado (diced)

1 tomato (diced)

Lime juice

Cilantro

Salt.

Instructions:

Bake sweet potatoes at 400°F until tender.

Mix black beans, avocado, tomato, lime juice, cilantro, and salt.

Top sweet potatoes with salsa.

Chicken Almond Salad

Ingredients:

4 oz cooked chicken breast (chopped)

¼ cup almonds (sliced)

1 apple (diced)

2 stalks celery (chopped)

2 tablespoons Greek yogurt

1 tablespoon Dijon mustard

Salt, and pepper

Instructions:

Mix chicken, almonds, apple, and celery.

In another bowl, combine Greek yogurt, mustard, salt, and pepper.

Combine all, chill before serving.

Zucchini Noodles with Pesto and Cherry Tomatoes

Ingredients:

2 zucchinis (spiraled)

1 cup cherry tomatoes (halved)

¼ cup pesto sauce

Parmesan cheese

Instructions:

Toss zucchini noodles with pesto.

Serve topped with cherry tomatoes and a sprinkle of Parmesan cheese.

Lentil Soup with Carrots and Celery

Ingredients:

1 cup lentils

2 carrots (diced)

2 stalks celery (diced)

1 onion (diced)

4 cups vegetable broth

1 teaspoon thyme

Olive oil

Salt, and pepper.

Instructions:

Sauté onions, carrots, and celery in olive oil.

Add lentils, broth, and thyme.

Simmer until lentils are tender.

Season with salt and pepper.

Eggplant and Tomato Bake

Ingredients:

1 eggplant (sliced)

2 tomatoes (sliced)

1 cup marinara sauce

½ cup mozzarella cheese

¼ cup basil leaves

Olive oil

Salt, and pepper.

Instructions:

Layer eggplant and tomato slices in a baking dish.

Top with marinara and mozzarella.

Bake at 375°F for 25 minutes. Garnish with basil.

DINNER RECIPES

DINNER RECIPES
Baked Salmon with Dill and Lemon

Ingredients:

4 salmon fillets

2 tablespoons olive oil

1 lemon (sliced)

Fresh dill

Salt, and pepper.

Instructions:

Place salmon on a baking sheet

Drizzle with olive oil

Season with salt and pepper.

Top with lemon slices and dill.

Bake at 375°F for 20 minutes.

Chicken and Vegetable Stir-Fry

Ingredients:

4 oz chicken breast (sliced)

2 cups mixed vegetables (bell peppers, broccoli, carrots)

2 tablespoons low-sodium soy sauce

1 tablespoon olive oil

1 garlic clove (minced)

Ginger.

Instructions:

Heat olive oil in a pan, add chicken and cook until browned.

Add vegetables, garlic, and ginger, stir-fry until tender.

Add soy sauce and cook for another minute.

Walnut-Crusted Cod

Ingredients:

4 cod fillets

½ cup walnuts (finely chopped)

1 tablespoon Dijon mustard

1 tablespoon olive oil

Lemon zest

Salt, and pepper.

Instructions:

Brush cod with mustard, press into chopped walnuts to coat.

Place on a baking sheet, drizzle with olive oil, season with

lemon zest, salt, and pepper.

Bake at 400°F for 12-15 minutes.

Roasted Chicken with Sweet Potatoes and Brussels Sprouts

Ingredients:

4 chicken thighs

2 sweet potatoes (cubed)

2 cups Brussels sprouts (halved)

2 tablespoons olive oil

Thyme

Salt, and pepper

Instructions:

Toss sweet potatoes and Brussels sprouts with olive oil, thyme, salt, and pepper.

Place chicken on top.

Roast at 425°F for 35-40 minutes.

Vegetarian Black Bean Chili

Ingredients:

2 cans black beans (drained)

1 can diced tomatoes

1 onion (diced)

1 bell pepper (diced)

2 garlic cloves (minced)

1 tablespoon chili powder

1 teaspoon cumin

Olive oil

Instructions:

Sauté onion, bell pepper, and garlic in olive oil.

Add beans, tomatoes, chili powder, and cumin.

Simmer for 30 minutes.

Season with salt and pepper.

Turmeric and Ginger Roasted Cauliflower

Ingredients:

1 head cauliflower (cut into florets)

2 tablespoons olive oil

1 teaspoon turmeric

½ teaspoon ground ginger

Salt, and pepper

Instructions:

Toss cauliflower with olive oil, turmeric, ginger, salt, and pepper.

Roast at 425°F for 25-30 minutes until golden and tender.

Baked Tilapia with Spinach and Tomatoes

Ingredients:

4 tilapia fillets

2 cups spinach

1 cup cherry tomatoes (halved)

1 garlic clove (minced)

2 tablespoons olive oil

Lemon juice

Salt, and pepper.

Instructions:

Place spinach and tomatoes in a baking dish, top with tilapia.

Season with garlic, lemon juice, salt, and pepper.

Drizzle with olive oil.

Bake at 375°F for 20 minutes.

Stuffed Bell Peppers with Ground Turkey and Veggies

Ingredients:

4 bell peppers (halved and seeded)

1 lb. ground turkey

1 cup chopped vegetables (zucchini, mushrooms)

1 can diced tomatoes

1 teaspoon oregano

1 garlic clove (minced)

Olive oil

Salt, and pepper

Instructions:

Sauté turkey, vegetables, garlic, oregano, salt, and pepper in olive oil until cooked.

Stir in tomatoes.

Stuff peppers with mixture.

Bake at 375°F for 30 minutes.

Lemon Garlic Shrimp with Asparagus

Ingredients:

1 lb. shrimp (peeled and deveined)

2 cups asparagus (trimmed)

2 tablespoons olive oil

3 garlic cloves (minced)

1 lemon (juice and zest)

Salt, and pepper

Instructions:

Heat olive oil in a pan, add garlic and asparagus.

Cook until tender.

Add shrimp, lemon juice, zest, salt, and pepper.

Cook until shrimp are pink.

Eggplant Lasagna

Ingredients:

2 eggplants (sliced lengthwise)

1 lb. ground beef or turkey

1 jar marinara sauce

1 cup ricotta cheese

1 cup shredded mozzarella

1 teaspoon oregano

Olive oil

Salt, and pepper

Instructions:

Grill eggplant slices until tender.

Cook meat, add marinara.

Layer eggplant, meat sauce, and cheeses in a baking dish, ending with mozzarella.

Bake at 375°F for 30 minutes.

SOUP RECIPE

SOUP RECIPE

Broccoli Almond Soup

Ingredients:

2 cups broccoli florets

1/4 cup ground almonds

1 onion (chopped)

2 cloves garlic (minced)

4 cups vegetable broth

1/2 cup almond milk

Olive oil

Salt, and pepper.

Instructions:

Sauté onion and garlic in olive oil until soft.

Add broccoli and broth; simmer until tender.

Blend until smooth

Stir in almond milk and ground almonds, season with salt and pepper.

Carrot Ginger Soup

Ingredients:

1 lb. carrots (chopped)

2 tablespoons fresh ginger (minced)

1 onion (chopped)

4 cups vegetable broth

1 cup coconut milk

Olive oil

Salt, and pepper

Instructions:

Sauté onion and ginger until fragrant.

Add carrots and broth; simmer until carrots are soft.

Blend until smooth

Stir in coconut milk

Season with salt and pepper.

Spinach and White Bean Soup

Ingredients:

1 can white beans (drained)

2 cups spinach

1 onion (chopped)

2 cloves garlic (minced)

4 cups vegetable broth

1 teaspoon thyme

Olive oil

Salt, and pepper

Instructions:

Sauté onion and garlic in olive oil.

Add beans, broth, and thyme; simmer for 15 minutes.

Add spinach, cook until wilted, season with salt and pepper.

Tomato Basil Soup

Ingredients:

4 cups ripe tomatoes (chopped)

1 onion (chopped)

2 cloves garlic (minced)

1/4 cup fresh basil (chopped)

3 cups vegetable broth

1/2 cup heavy cream

Olive oil

Salt, and pepper

Instructions:

Sauté onion and garlic.

Add tomatoes and broth; simmer for 20 minutes.

Blend until smooth, return to pot

Stir in cream and basil

Season with salt and pepper.

Chicken and Vegetable Soup

Ingredients:

1 lb. chicken breast (cubed)

2 carrots (chopped)

2 celery stalks (chopped)

1 onion (chopped)

4 cups chicken broth

1 teaspoon rosemary

Olive oil

Salt, and pepper

Instructions:

Sauté chicken until browned.

Add vegetables and cook until soft.

Add broth and rosemary.

Simmer until chicken is cooked through.

Season with salt and pepper.

Mushroom and Barley Soup

Ingredients:

1 lb. mushrooms (sliced)

1 cup barley

1 onion (chopped)

2 cloves garlic (minced)

6 cups vegetable broth

1 teaspoon thyme

Olive oil

Salt, and pepper

Instructions:

Sauté onion, garlic, and mushrooms.

Add broth, barley, and thyme.

Simmer until barley is tender.

Season with salt and pepper.

Roasted Red Pepper and Lentil Soup

Ingredients:

1 lb. red lentils

2 red bell peppers (roasted and peeled)

1 onion (chopped)

2 cloves garlic (minced)

6 cups vegetable broth

1 teaspoon smoked paprika

Olive oil

Salt, and pepper

Instructions:

Sauté onion and garlic.

Add lentils, roasted peppers, broth, and paprika.

Simmer until lentils are soft.

Blend until smooth, season with salt and pepper.

Cauliflower and Leek Soup

Ingredients:

1 head cauliflower (chopped)

2 leeks (cleaned and sliced)

4 cups vegetable broth

1 cup heavy cream

Olive oil

Salt, and pepper

Instructions:

Sauté leeks until soft.

Add cauliflower and broth; simmer until tender.

Blend until smooth, stir in cream

Season with salt and pepper.

Butternut Squash and Apple Soup

Ingredients:

1 butternut squash (peeled and cubed)

2 apples (peeled and chopped)

1 onion (chopped)

4 cups vegetable broth

1 teaspoon cinnamon

1/2 cup coconut milk

Olive oil

Salt, and pepper

Instructions:

Sauté onion until translucent.

Add squash, apples, broth, and cinnamon.

Simmer until squash is soft.

Blend until smooth, stir in coconut milk.

Season with salt and pepper.

Sweet Potato and Sage Soup

Ingredients:

2 sweet potatoes (peeled and cubed)

1 onion (chopped)

2 cloves garlic (minced)

4 cups vegetable broth

1 tablespoon fresh sage (chopped)

1/2 cup heavy cream

Olive oil

Salt, and pepper

Instructions:

Sauté onion and garlic.

Add sweet potatoes, broth, and sage

Simmer until potatoes are tender.

Blend until smooth, stir in cream

Season with salt and pepper.

SNACKS RECIPE

SNACKS RECIPE

Avocado Toast with Cherry Tomatoes

Ingredients:

1 ripe avocado

2 slices of whole-grain bread

½ cup cherry tomatoes (halved)

Lemon juice

Salt, and pepper

Instructions:

Mash the avocado and mix with a bit of lemon juice, salt, and pepper.

Spread on toasted bread and top with cherry tomatoes.

Blueberry Yogurt Parfait

Ingredients:

1 cup Greek yogurt,

½ cup fresh blueberries,

¼ cup granola,

1 tablespoon honey.

Instructions:

Layer Greek yogurt, blueberries, and granola in a glass.

Drizzle with honey.

Cucumber and Hummus Cups

Ingredients:

1 large cucumber (sliced into thick rounds)

1 cup hummus

Paprika

Fresh parsley

Instructions

Scoop a small portion from the top of each cucumber slice to form a cup.

Fill with hummus, sprinkle with paprika, and garnish with parsley.

Apple Peanut Butter Slices

Ingredients:

1 apple (cored and sliced)

¼ cup natural peanut butter

1 tablespoon slivered almonds

Cinnamon.

Instructions:

Spread peanut butter over apple slices.

Sprinkle with slivered almonds and a dash of cinnamon.

Carrot and Celery Sticks with Almond Butter

Ingredients:

2 carrots (peeled and cut into sticks)

2 celery stalks (cut into sticks)

¼ cup almond butter

Instructions:

Serve carrot and celery sticks with almond butter for dipping.

Baked Kale Chips

Ingredients:

1 bunch kale (torn into bite-sized pieces)

1 tablespoon olive oil

Salt.

Instructions:

Massage kale with olive oil and a pinch of salt.

Bake at 300°F (150°C) for 10-15 minutes until crisp.

Roasted Chickpeas

Ingredients:

1 can chickpeas (drained and rinsed)

1 tablespoon olive oil

½ teaspoon smoked paprika

Salt

Instructions:

Toss chickpeas with olive oil, paprika, and salt.

Roast at 425°F (220°C) for 20-30 minutes until crunchy.

Walnut-Stuffed Dates

Ingredients:

10 Medjool dates (pitted)

10 walnuts.

Instructions:

Insert a walnut into each date where the pit was removed.

Chia Seed Pudding

Ingredients:

¼ cup chia seeds,

1 cup almond milk,

1 tablespoon maple syrup,

½ teaspoon vanilla extract.

Instructions:

Mix all ingredients in a bowl.

Refrigerate overnight or until the pudding thickens.

Stir before serving.

Cheese and Grape Skewers

Ingredients:

20 grapes

20 cubes of cheese (such as cheddar or mozzarella)

10 skewers.

Instructions:

Alternate threading grapes and cheese cubes onto skewers.

CONCLUSION

"Mind Diet Cookbook," we embarked on a journey not just through the culinary arts but through the compassionate understanding of Alzheimer's disease and its impact on individuals and their families. Our goal was to offer more than just recipes; we aimed to provide a guide that enriches the lives of those affected by Alzheimer's through nutritious, brain-healthy foods that cater to their unique dietary needs.

Throughout the chapters, from breakfasts to dinners, soups to snacks, we meticulously selected ingredients known for their beneficial properties in supporting cognitive health and overall well-being. We avoided complex grains like quinoa to ensure that each recipe remains accessible, easy to digest, and enjoyable for everyone, especially considering the diverse dietary preferences and needs that may accompany Alzheimer's disease.

As we conclude this culinary journey, we hope that "The Alzheimer's Disease Cookbook" serves as a valuable tool in your kitchen, offering recipes that are both healthful and delightful. May it inspire you to create meals that comfort, nourish, and bring joy to both those living with Alzheimer's and their loved ones.

DAILY MEAL PLANNER

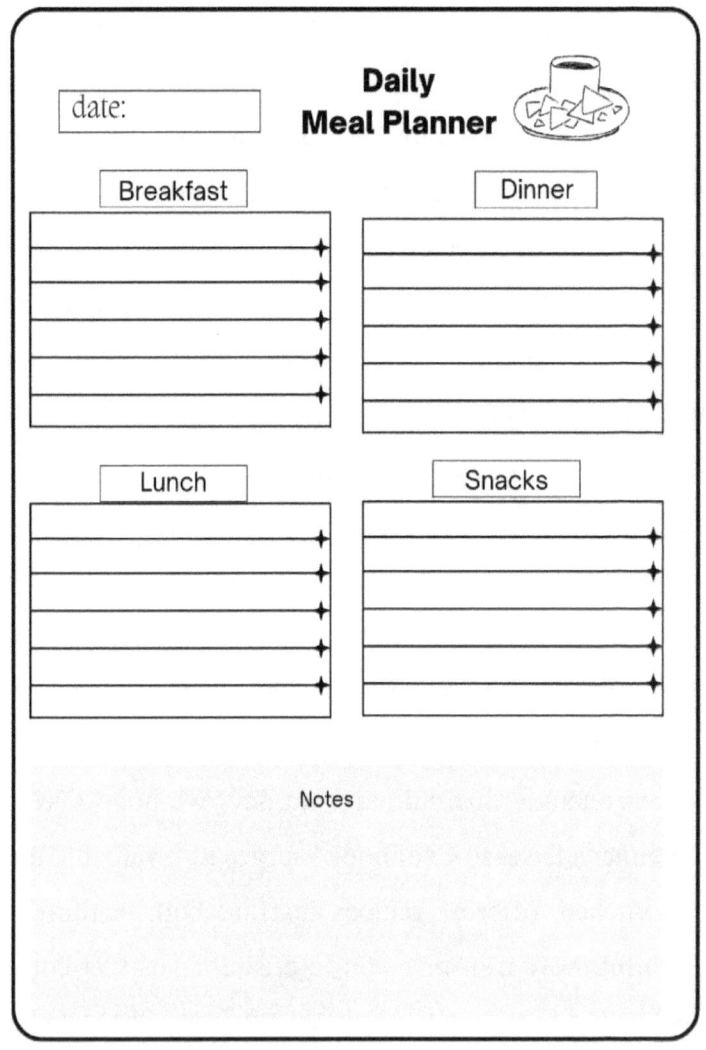

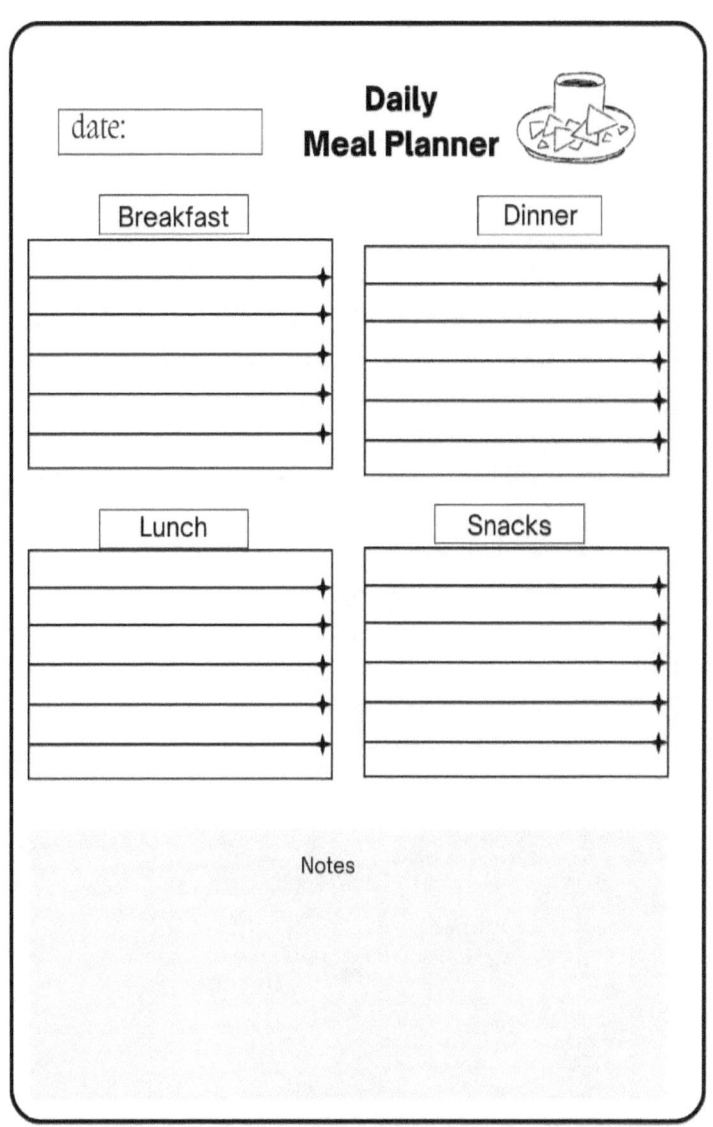

date:

Daily
Meal Planner

Breakfast

Dinner

Lunch

Snacks

Notes

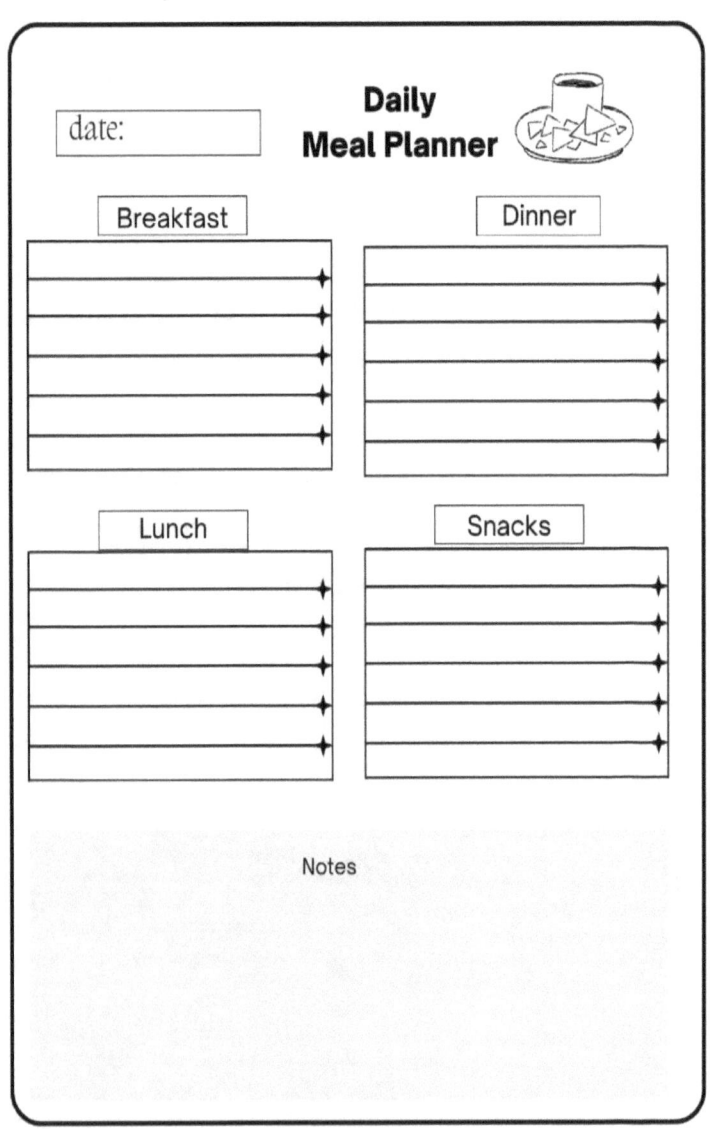

Daily
Meal Planner

date:

Breakfast

Dinner

Lunch

Snacks

Notes

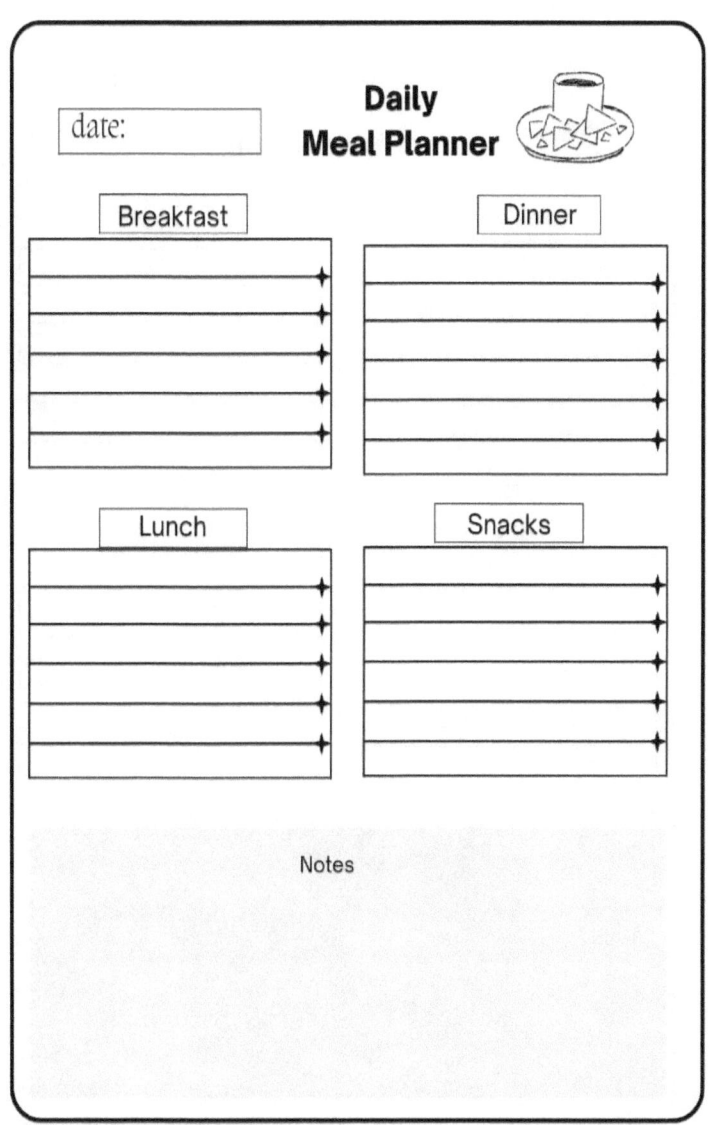

Daily
Meal Planner

date:

Breakfast

Dinner

Lunch

Snacks

Notes

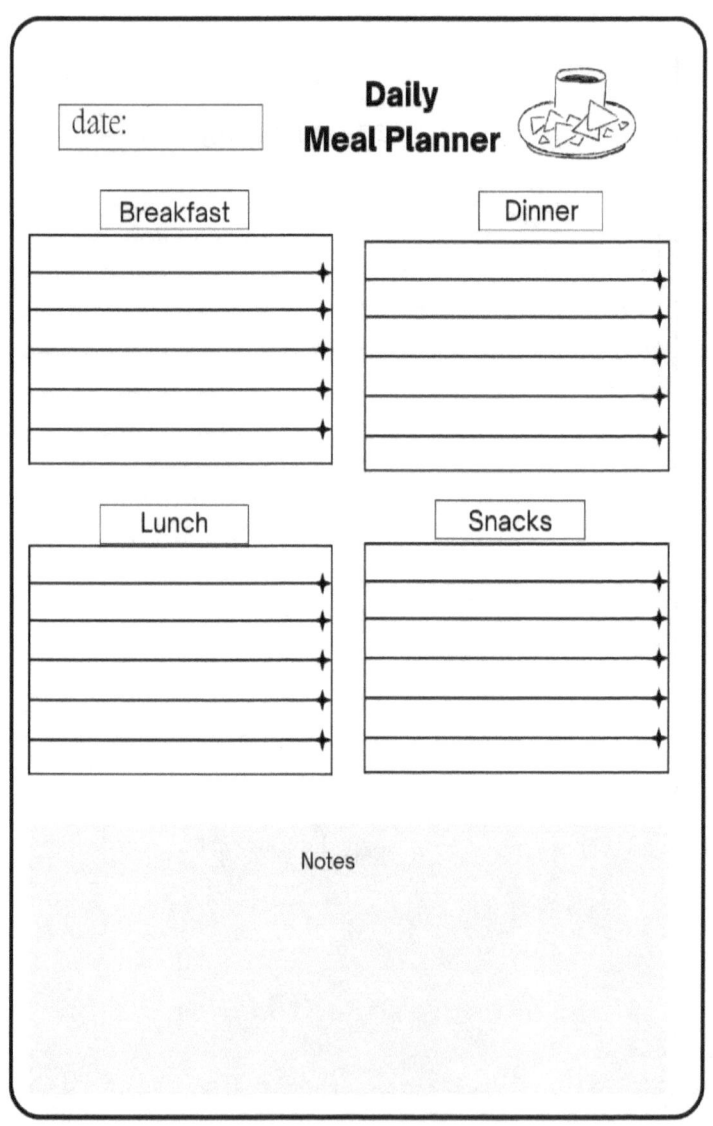

Daily Meal Planner

date:

Breakfast

Dinner

Lunch

Snacks

Notes

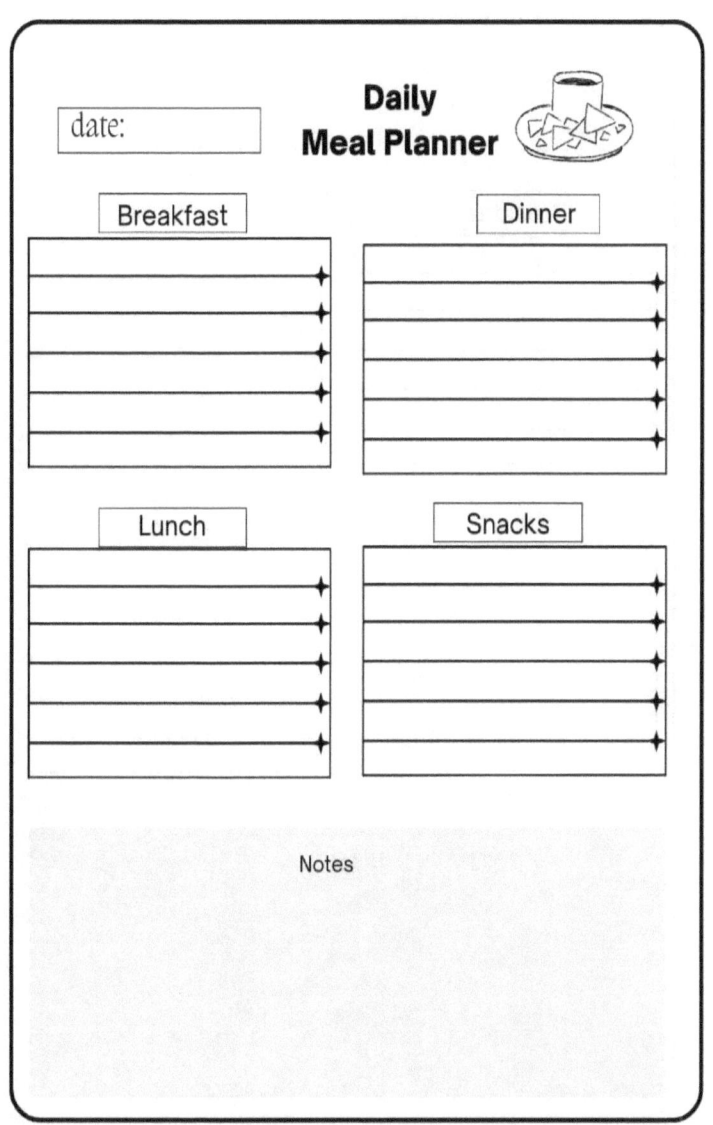

date:

Daily
Meal Planner

Breakfast

Dinner

Lunch

Snacks

Notes

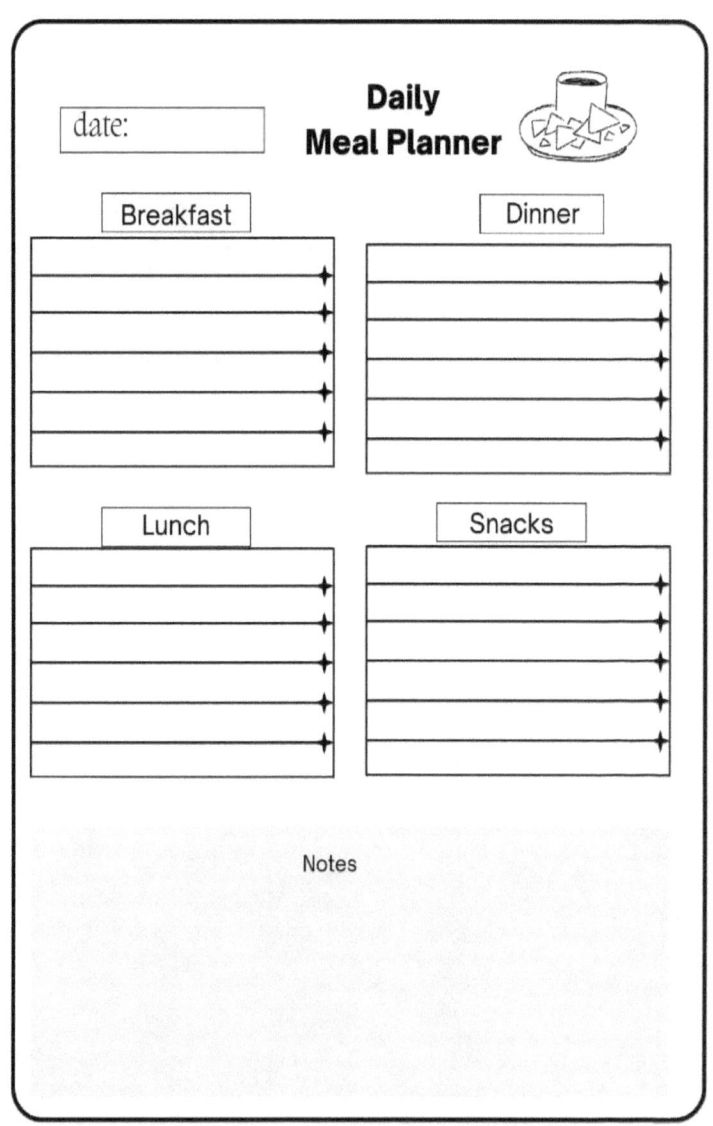

date:

Daily
Meal Planner

Breakfast

Dinner

Lunch

Snacks

Notes

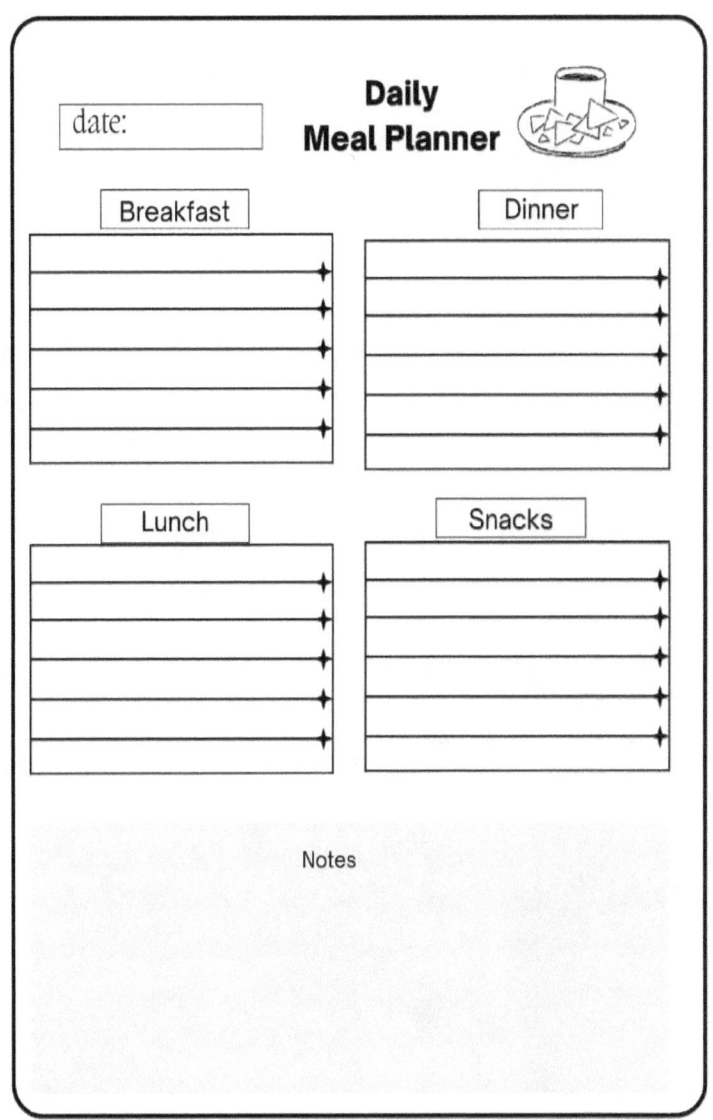

Daily Meal Planner

date:

Breakfast

Dinner

Lunch

Snacks

Notes

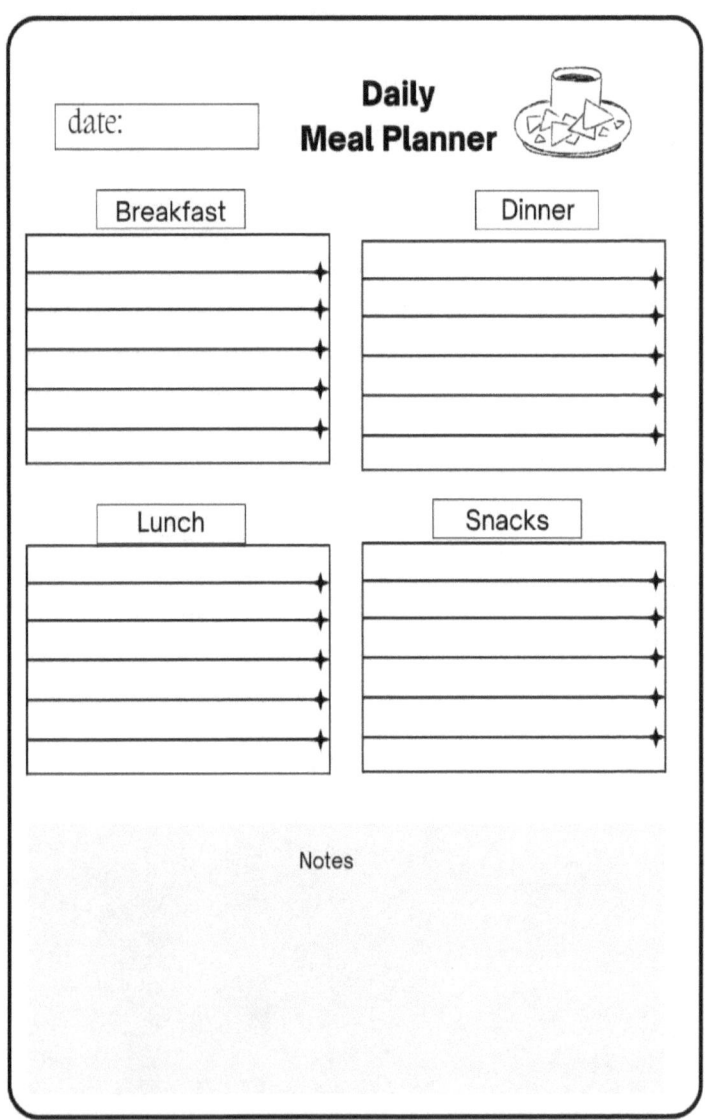

date:

**Daily
Meal Planner**

Breakfast

Dinner

Lunch

Snacks

Notes

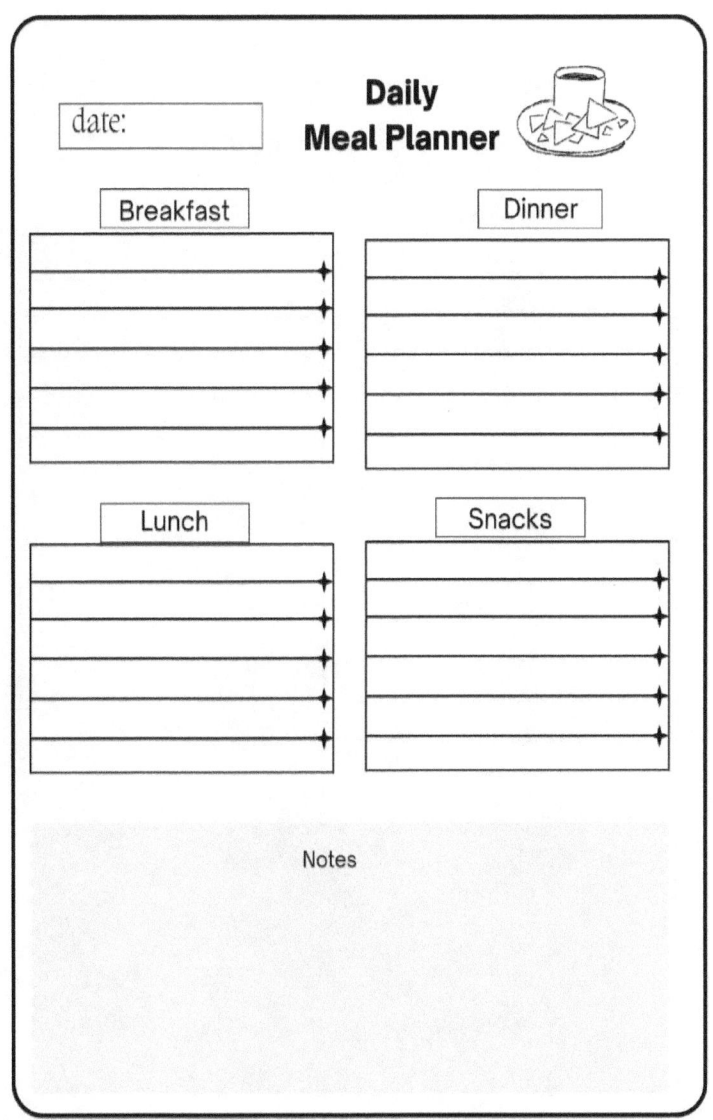

Daily Meal Planner

date:

Breakfast

Dinner

Lunch

Snacks

Notes

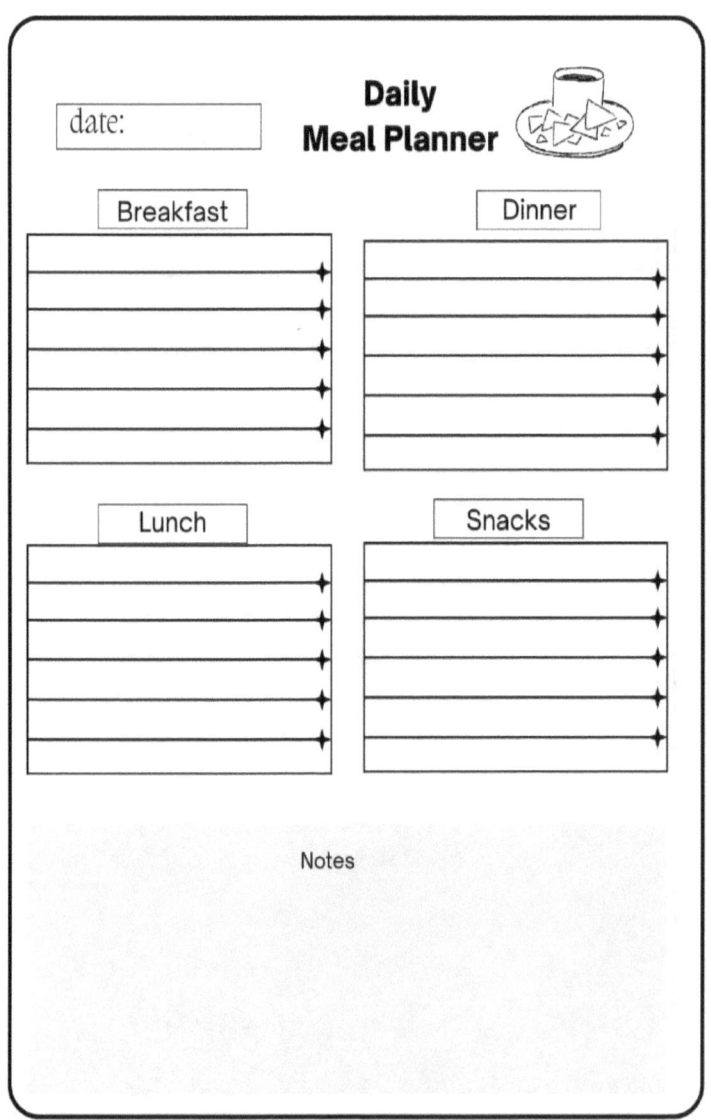

date:

Daily
Meal Planner

Breakfast

Dinner

Lunch

Snacks

Notes

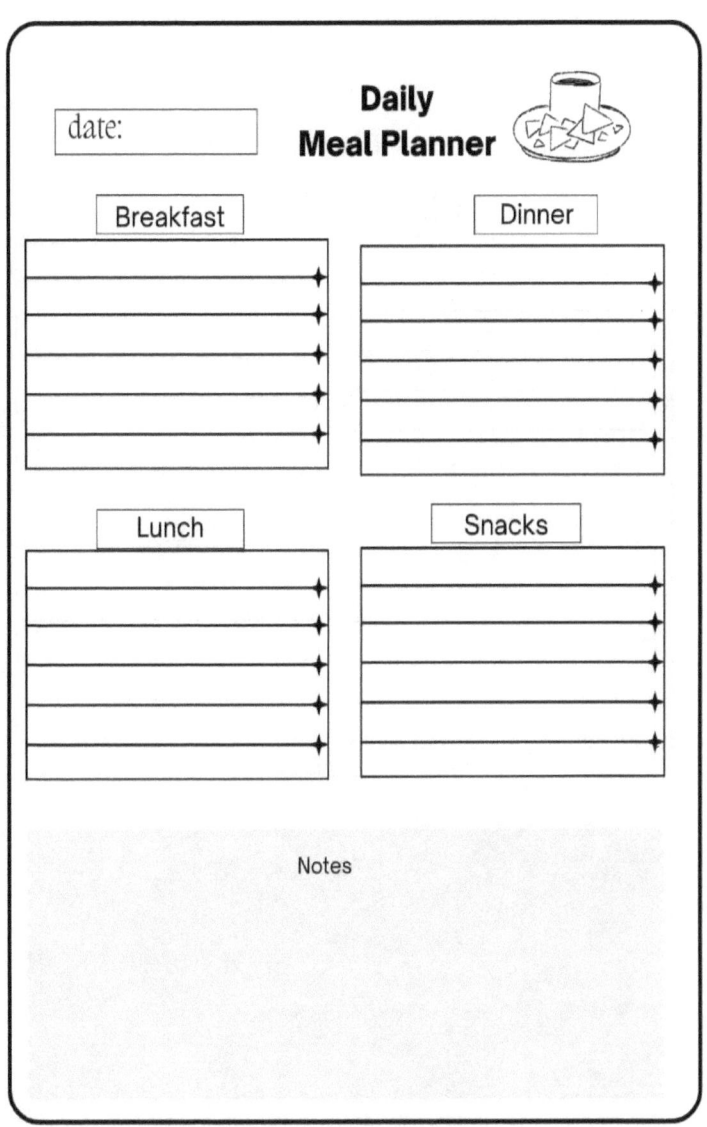

date:

Daily
Meal Planner

Breakfast

Dinner

Lunch

Snacks

Notes

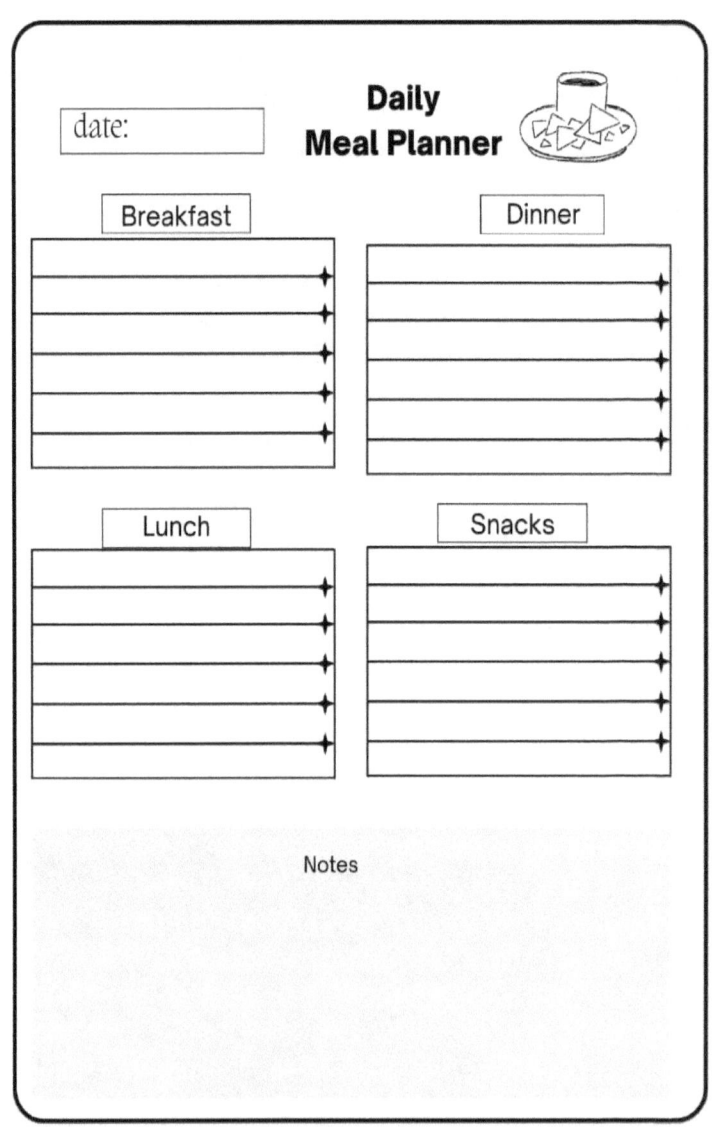

Daily Meal Planner

date:

Breakfast

Dinner

Lunch

Snacks

Notes

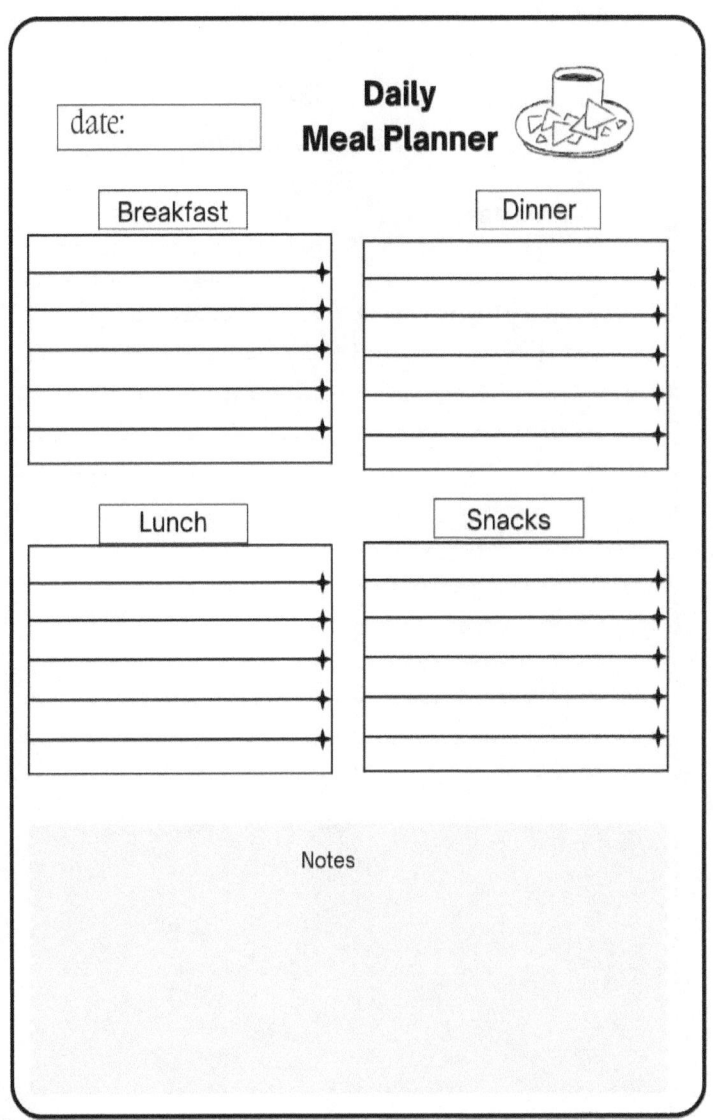

Daily
Meal Planner

date:

Breakfast

Dinner

Lunch

Snacks

Notes

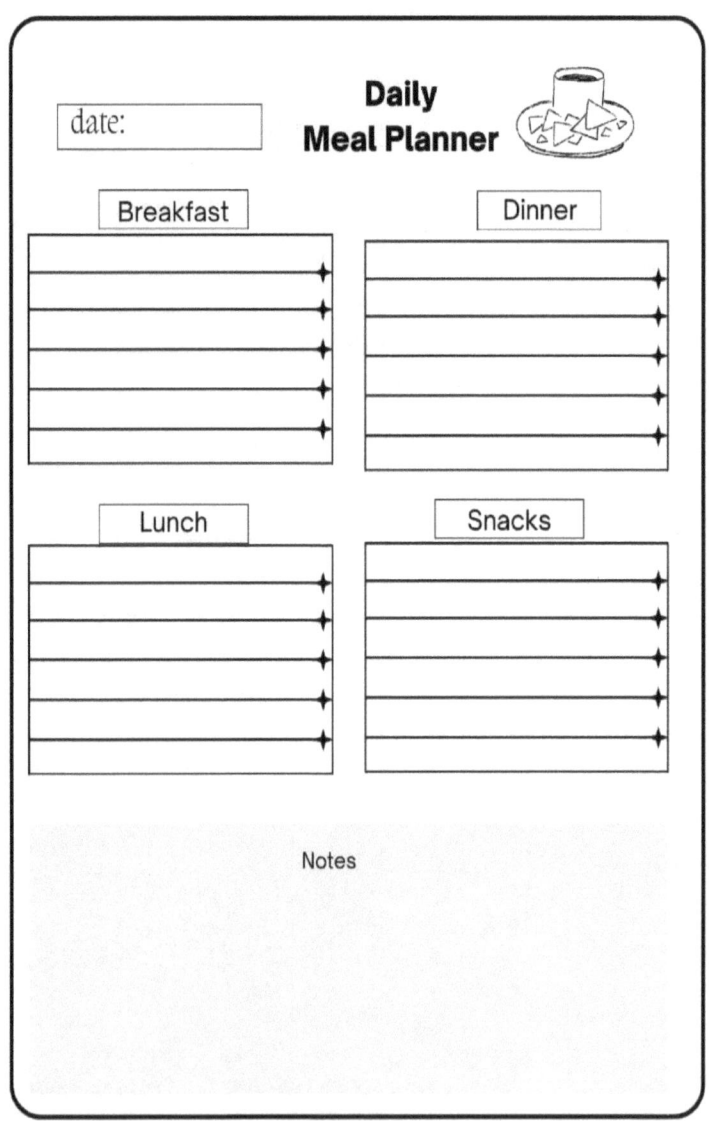

Daily Meal Planner

date:

Breakfast

Dinner

Lunch

Snacks

Notes

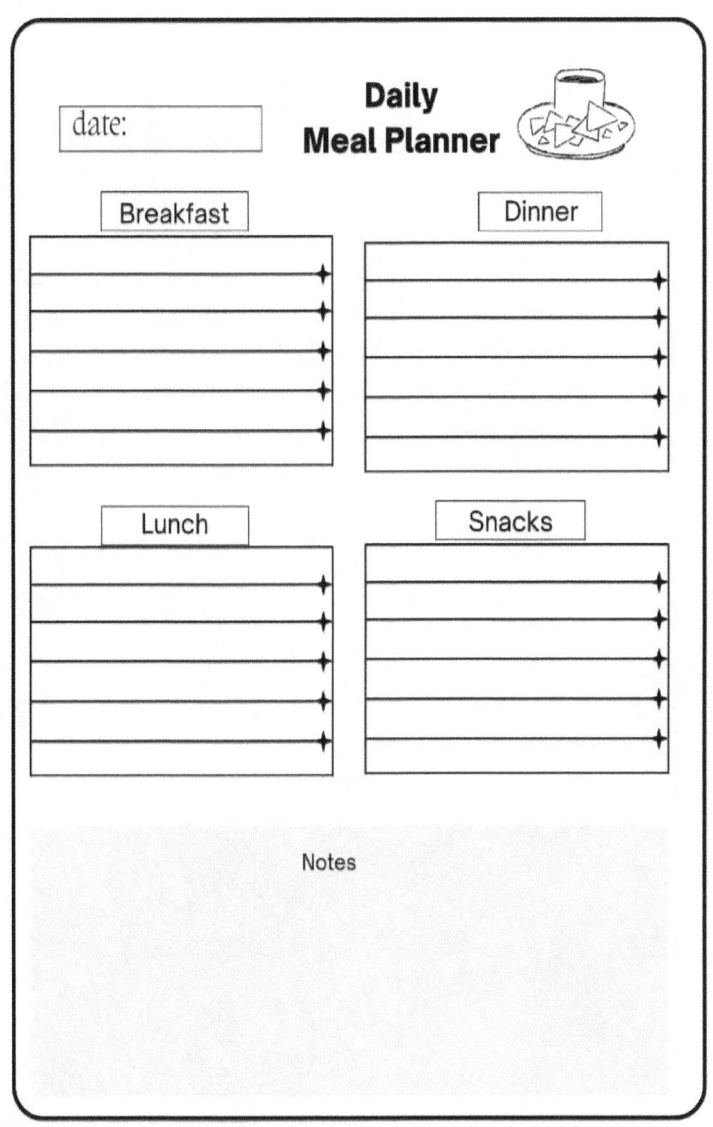

Daily
Meal Planner

date:

Breakfast

Dinner

Lunch

Snacks

Notes

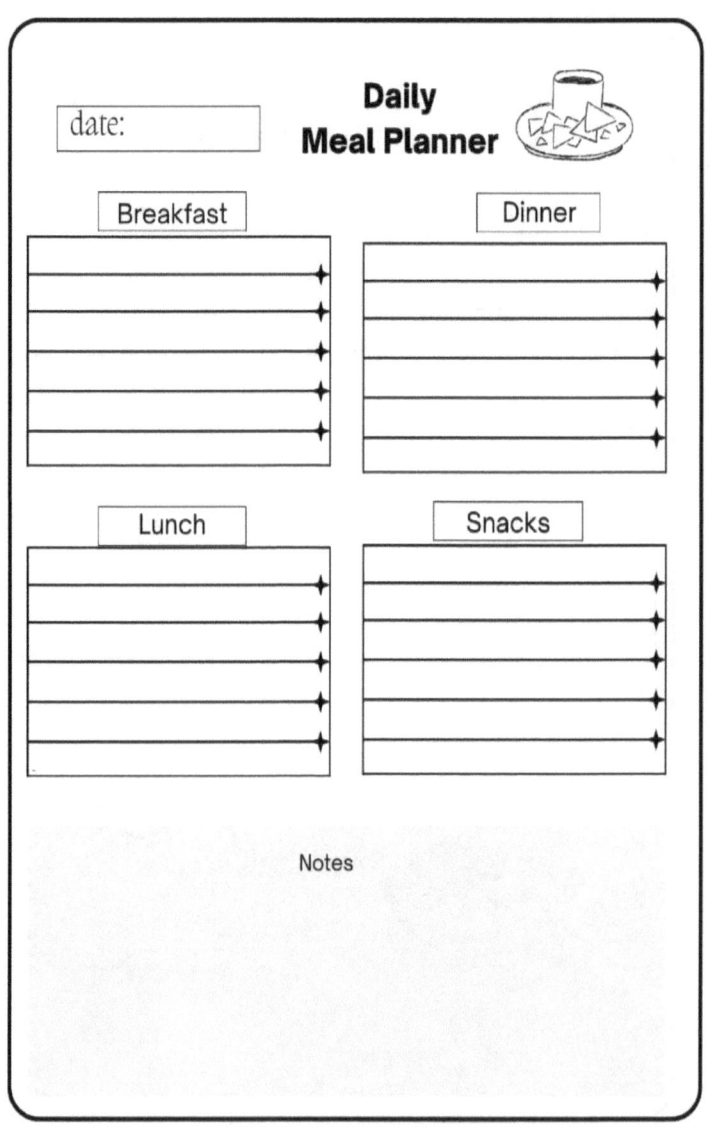

Daily Meal Planner

date:

Breakfast

Dinner

Lunch

Snacks

Notes

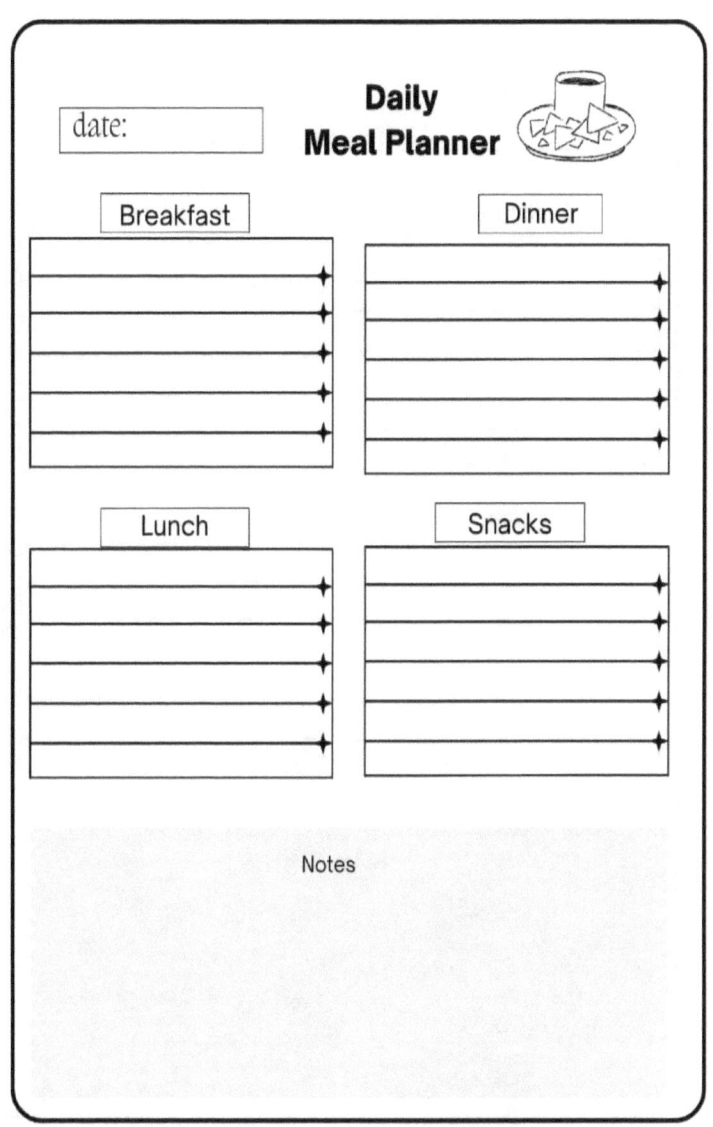

date:

**Daily
Meal Planner**

Breakfast

Dinner

Lunch

Snacks

Notes

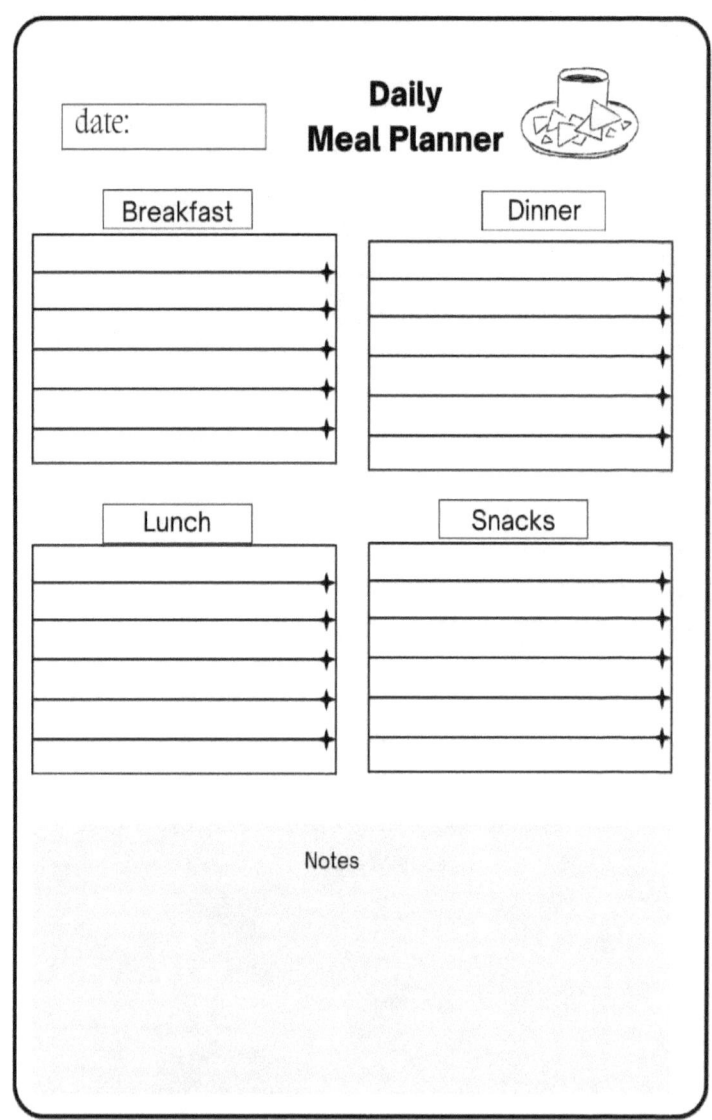

date:

Daily
Meal Planner

Breakfast

Dinner

Lunch

Snacks

Notes

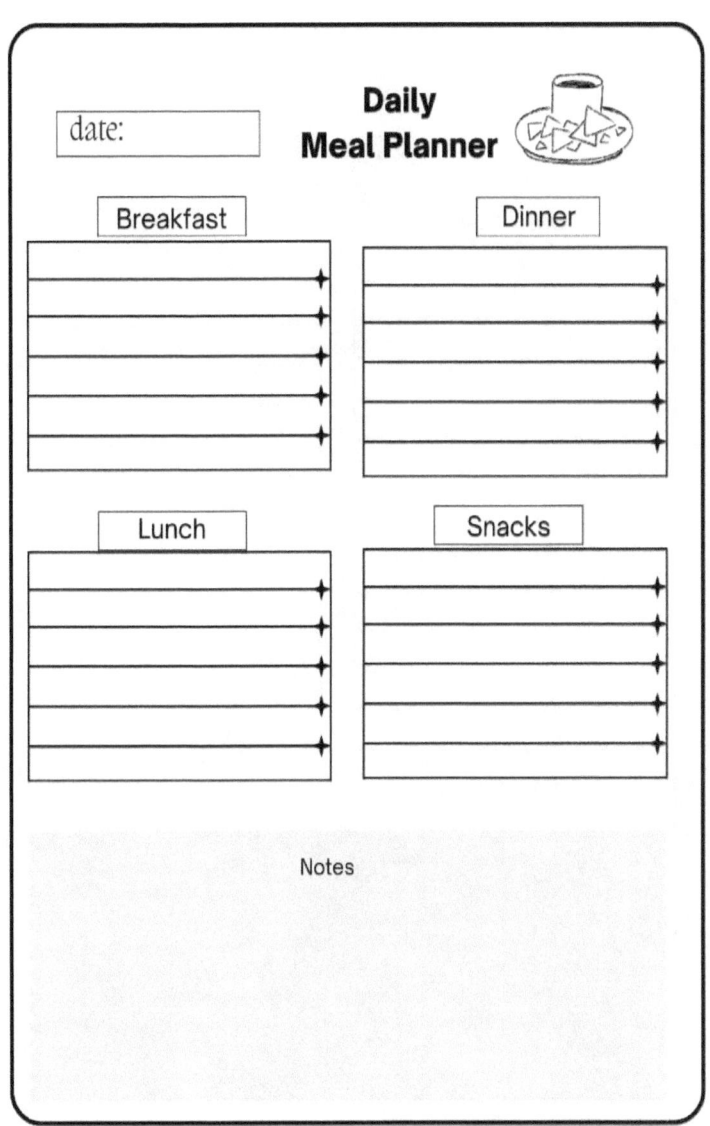

date:

Daily Meal Planner

Breakfast

Dinner

Lunch

Snacks

Notes

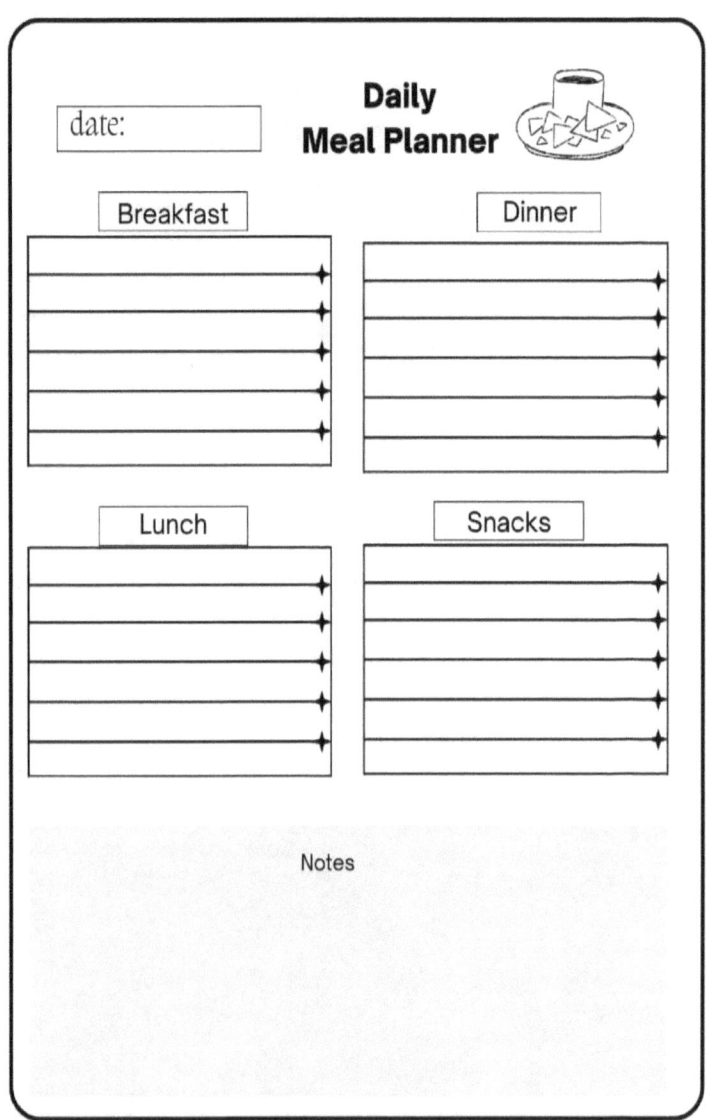

date:

**Daily
Meal Planner**

Breakfast

Dinner

Lunch

Snacks

Notes

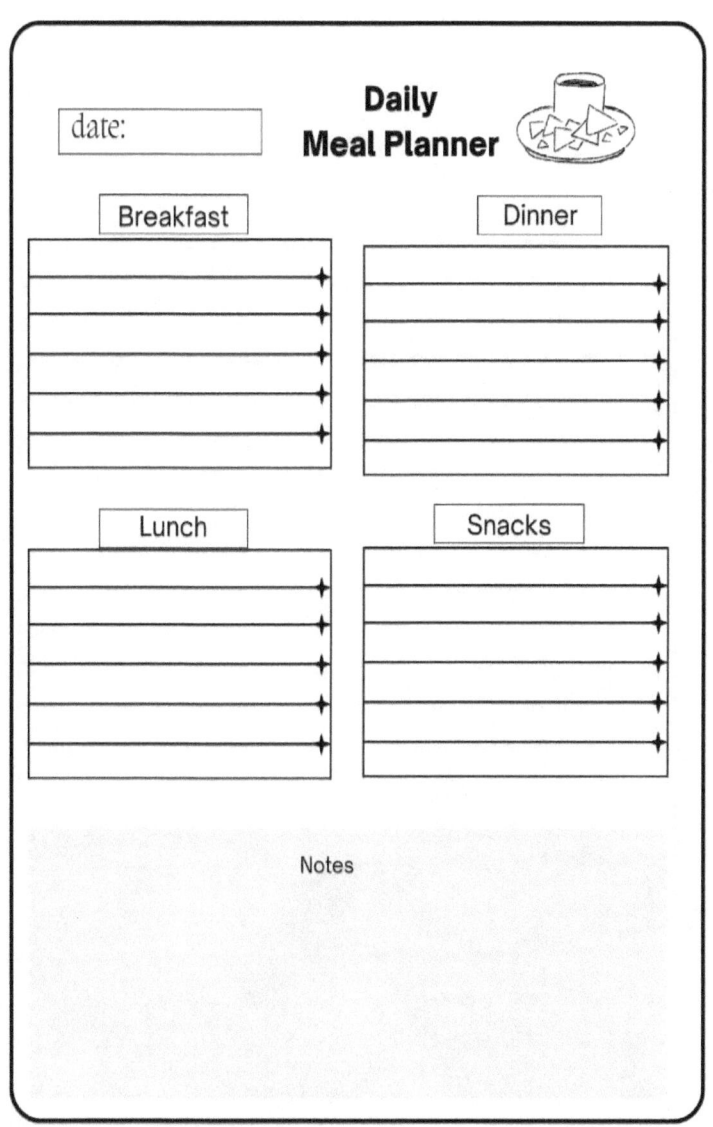

date:

Daily
Meal Planner

Breakfast

Dinner

Lunch

Snacks

Notes

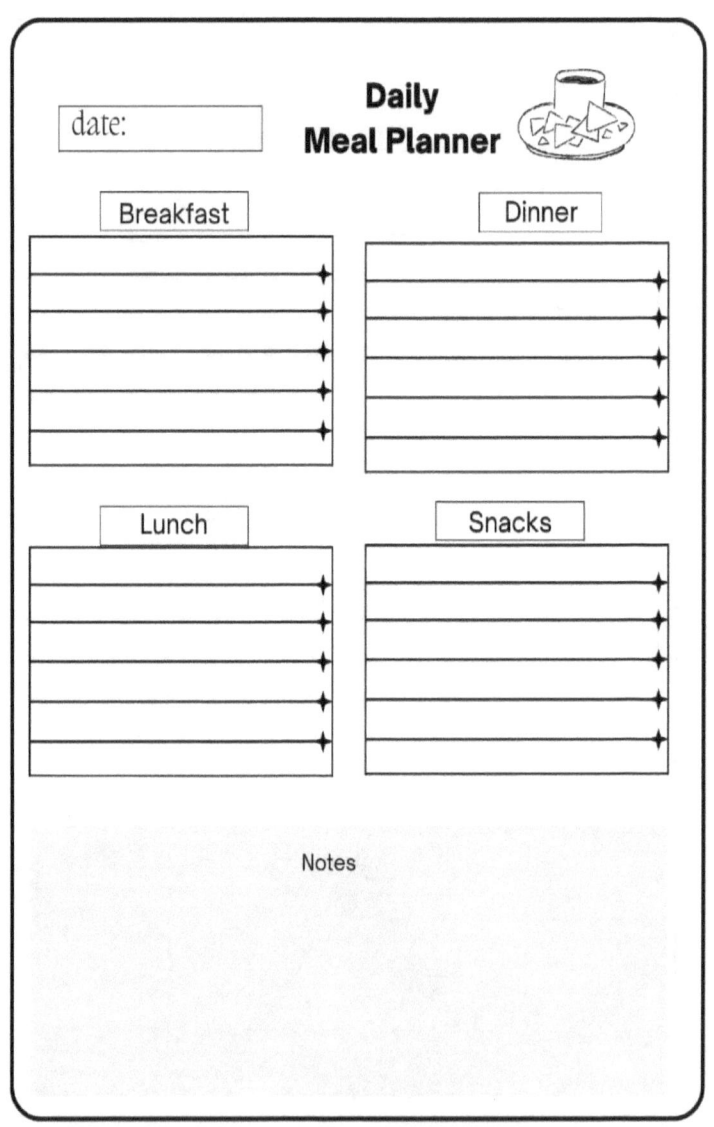

Daily Meal Planner

date:

Breakfast

Dinner

Lunch

Snacks

Notes

vv

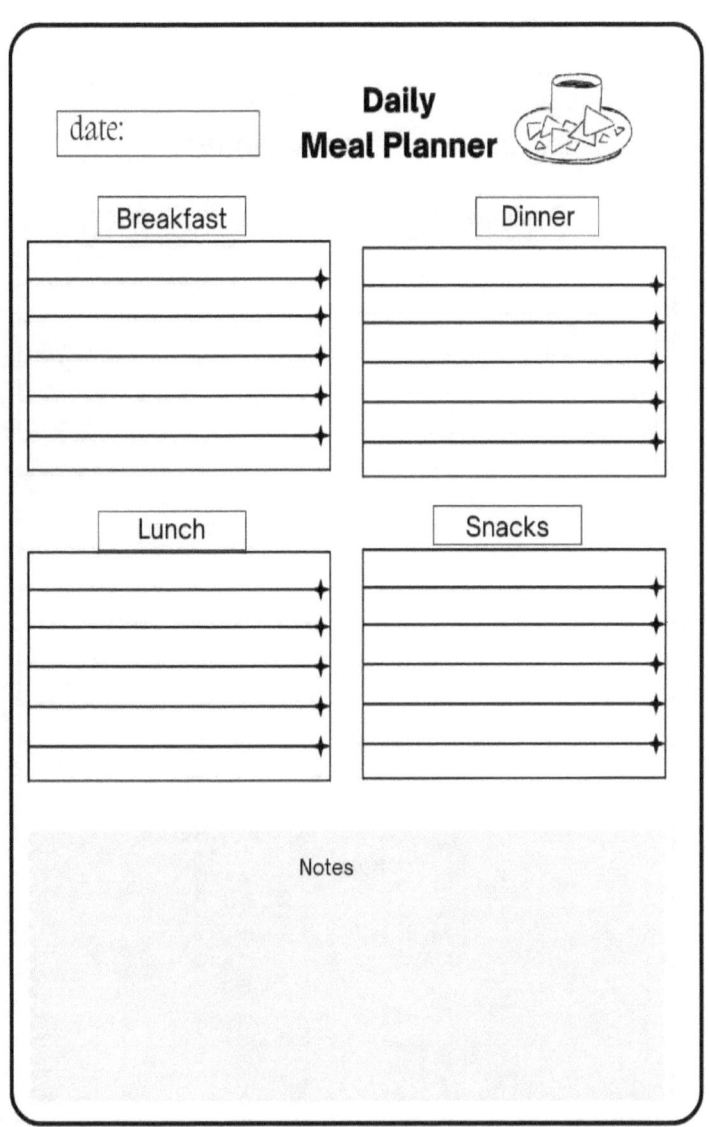

**Daily
Meal Planner**

date:

Breakfast

Dinner

Lunch

Snacks

Notes

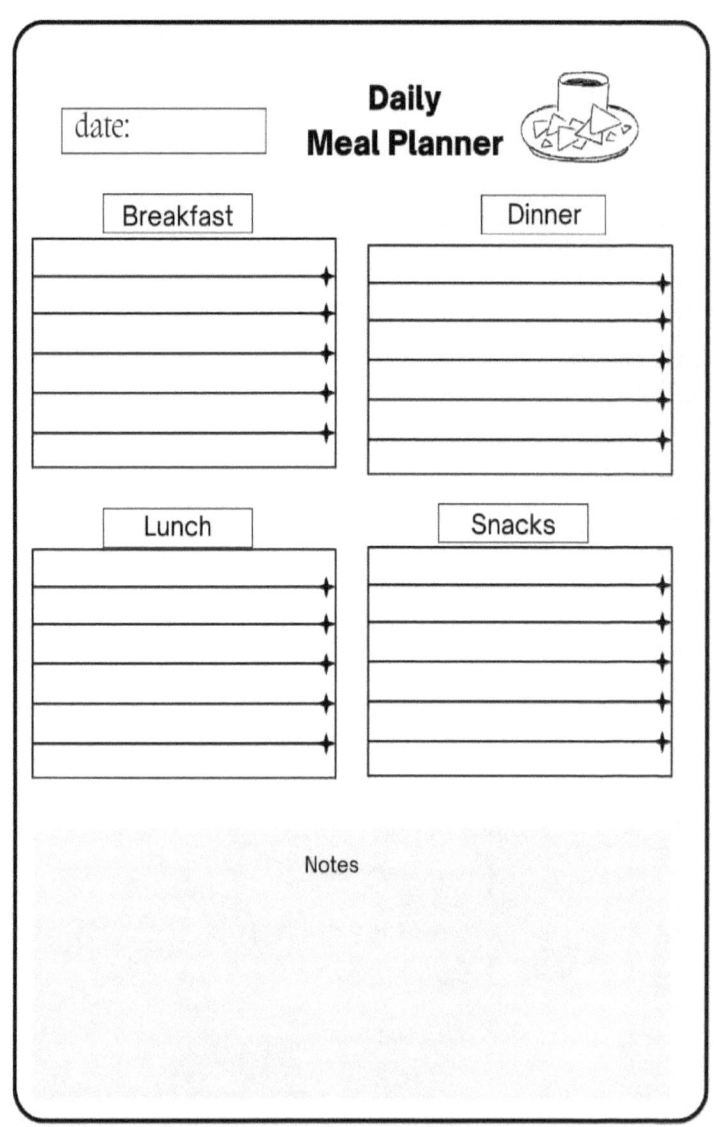

Daily
Meal Planner

date:

Breakfast

Dinner

Lunch

Snacks

Notes

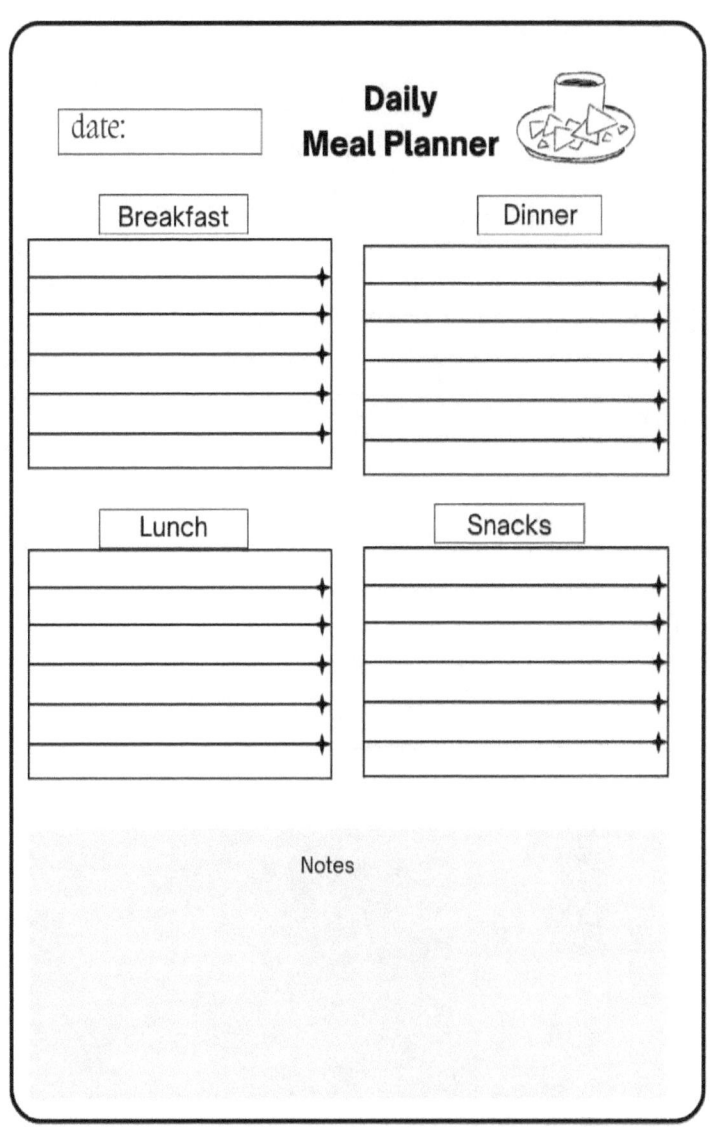

Daily
Meal Planner

date:

Breakfast

Dinner

Lunch

Snacks

Notes

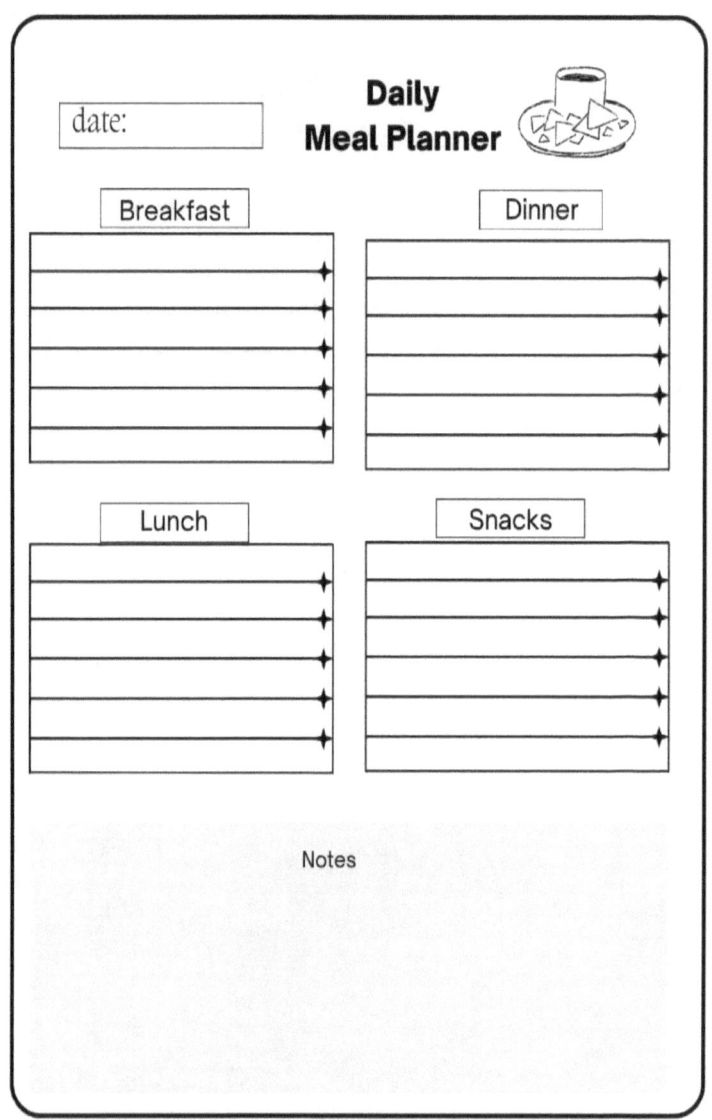

date:

Daily
Meal Planner

Breakfast

Dinner

Lunch

Snacks

Notes

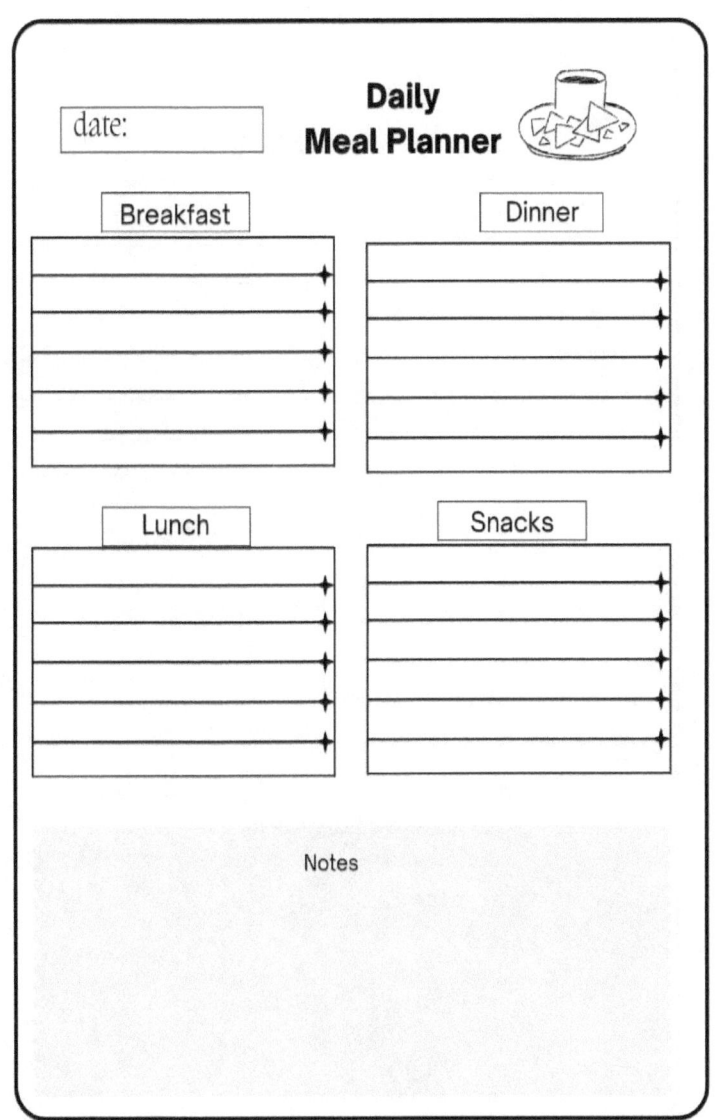

Daily
Meal Planner

date:

Breakfast

Dinner

Lunch

Snacks

Notes

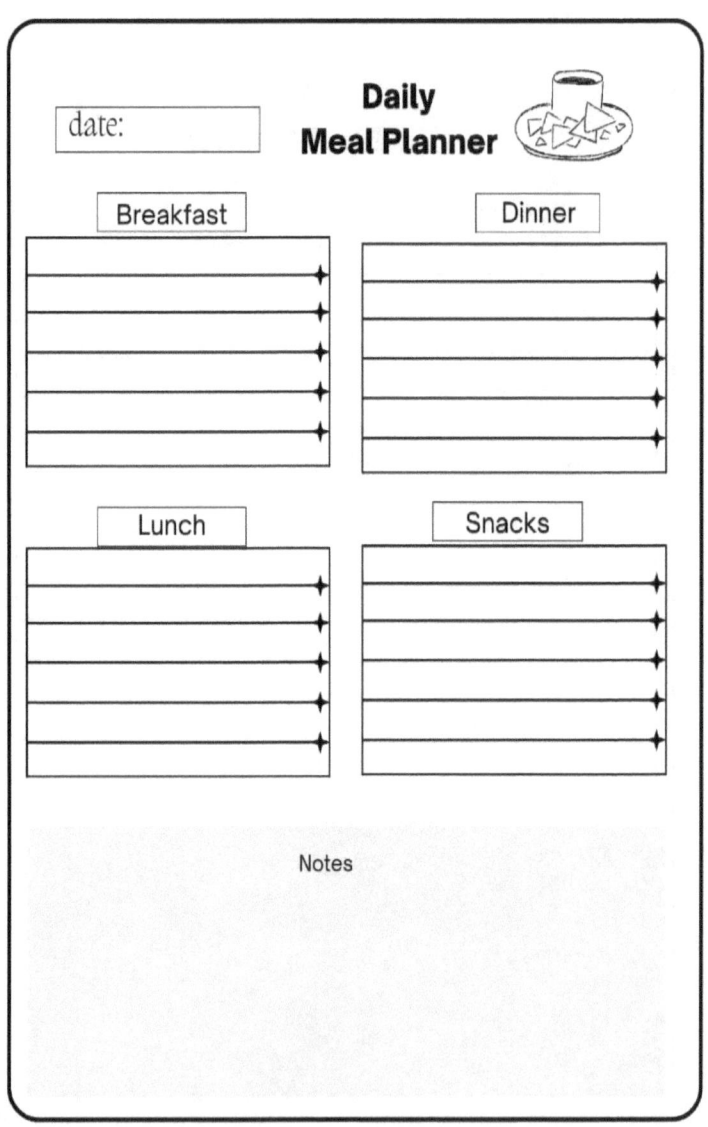

Daily
Meal Planner

date:

Breakfast

Dinner

Lunch

Snacks

Notes

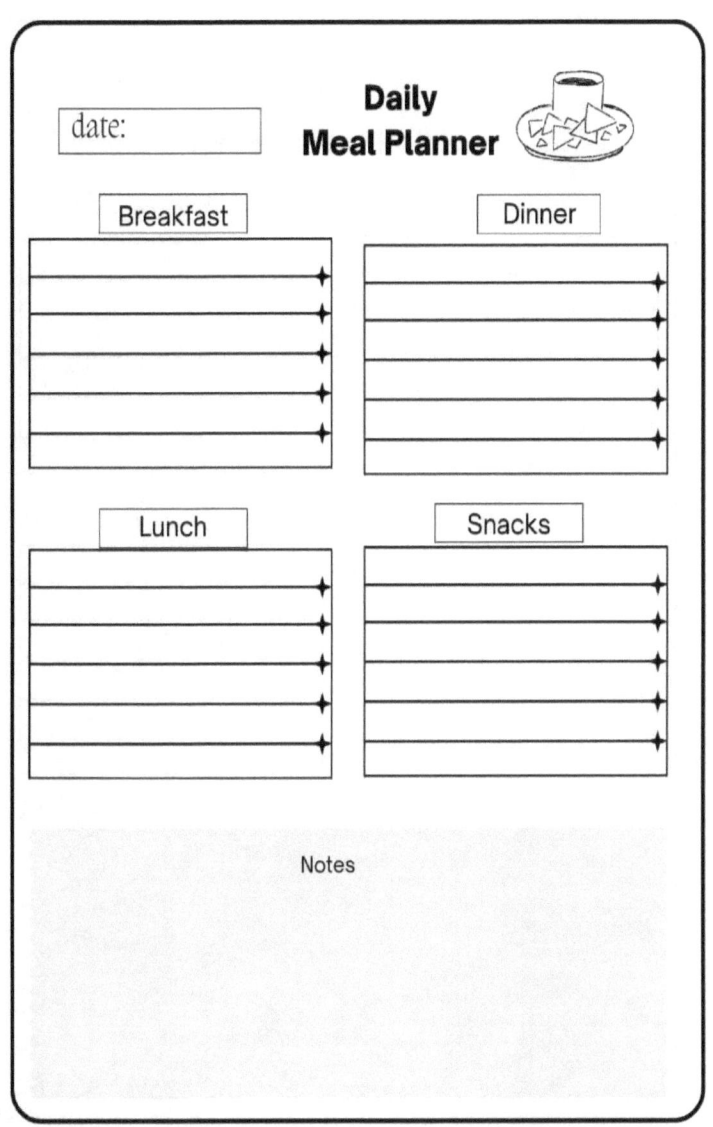

date:

Daily
Meal Planner

Breakfast

Dinner

Lunch

Snacks

Notes

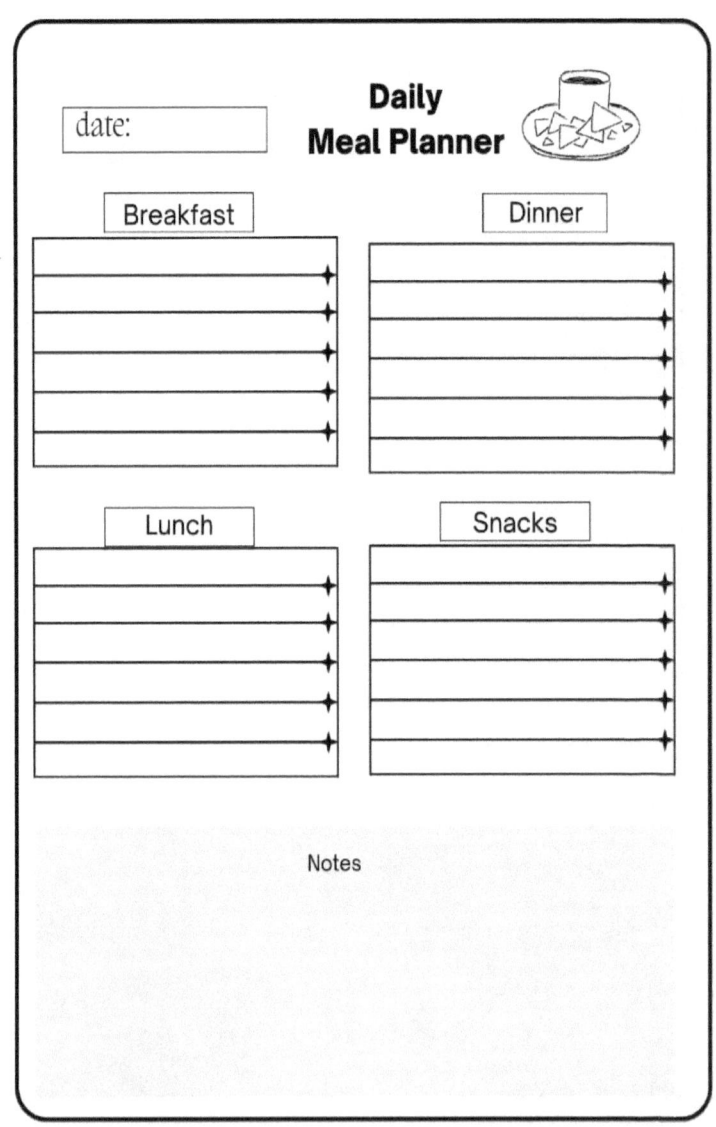

date:

**Daily
Meal Planner**

Breakfast

Dinner

Lunch

Snacks

Notes

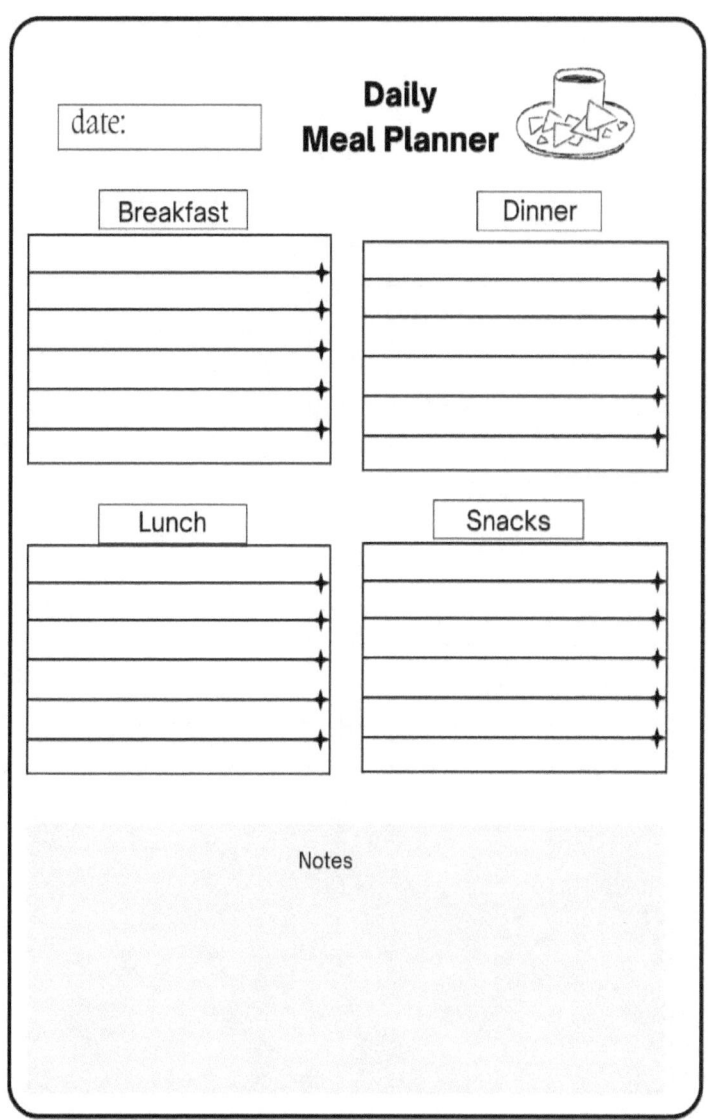

date:

Daily
Meal Planner

Breakfast

Dinner

Lunch

Snacks

Notes

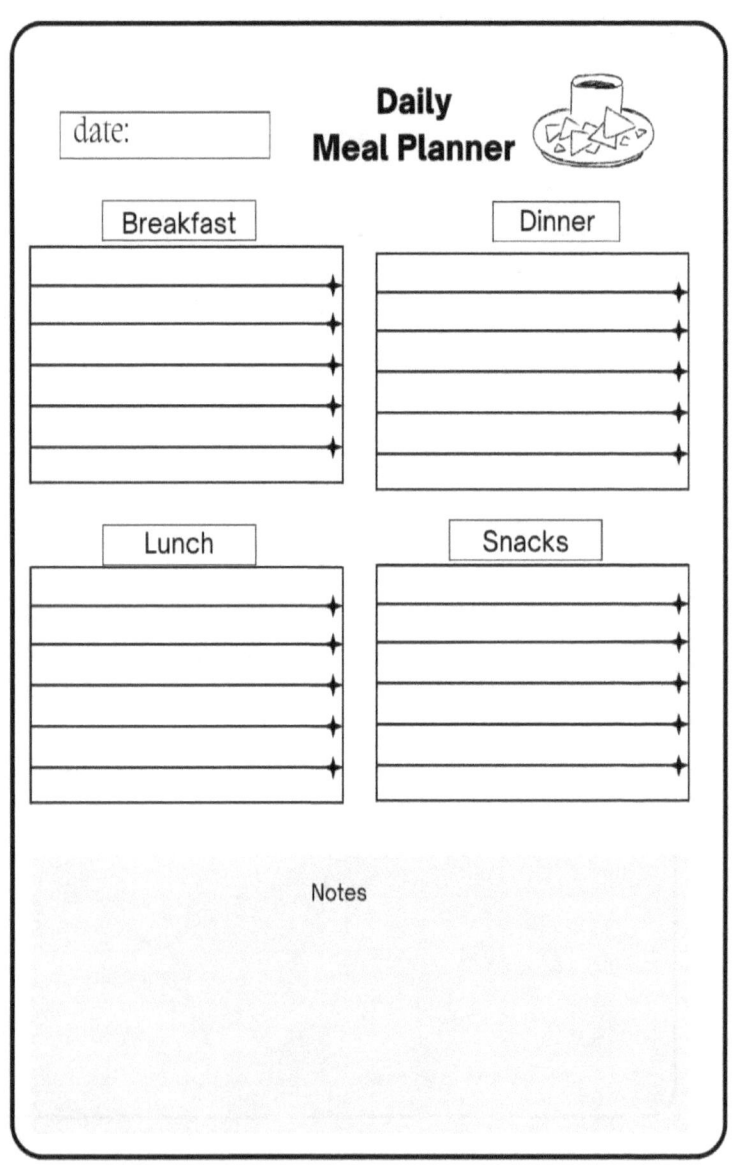

date:

**Daily
Meal Planner**

| Breakfast |
| Dinner |

| Lunch |
| Snacks |

Notes